Oil Pulling For Beginners

Oil Pulling Therapy -
The All Natural Remedy
For Oral Health, Combating Tooth Decay,
Gum Disease And Detoxifying Your Body
Through Oral Cleansing Using
Coconut Oil And Ayurvedic Methods

By: Ashley Stone

Table of Contents

Introduction

Oil Pulling has become an extremely fast growing phenomenon in western society. With a shifting focus on natural remedies and removal of toxins in our daily routine it is no wonder this ancient process has begun to gain so much traction.

"Oil Pulling For Beginners" contains a step by step guide to oil pulling as well as focussing on the many health benefits associated with the process. I know this book will add tremendous value to your life and I am really happy to know that I can help you on your journey towards a happy, healthy and all natural life!

Thank you again for downloading this book, I know you enjoy it!!

- Ashley Stone

Chapter 1
Sticks, Stones and Oil Pulling

A Very Human Problem

Some health fads come and go, while some go on for ever. Oil pulling is one of those healthy habits that has been with us for centuries – probably thousands of years. Since man, woman and child climbed down from the trees first hunting and gathering, and later learning to farm, one problem has needed solving: how to maintain a healthy mouth! Techniques have varied throughout the ages, some tried sticks and others tried stones (albeit finely ground ones). Others tried what we now know as oil pulling. It's a technique that goes back a long way, deeply rooted in Ayurvedic traditions from India and it's a very simple solution to the age old problem of how to maintain a healthy mouth full of shining white teeth.

Tooth decay and disease is a very human problem; from cavities to tooth loss through to painful, damaging tooth disease. We are often told that we are what we eat and it's certainly true that what we eat can have a profound affect on our weight, health and lifespan. A healthy mouth and healthy teeth are both essential to ensuring that we can get the right fuel for our bodies into it in the first place.

Our bodies do a lot of the hard work for us when it comes to keeping our mouths healthy; saliva is naturally antiseptic and helps to heal injuries in the mouth. Bacteria and micro-organisms also occur naturally in our mouths and are also swallowed and taken into the gut. Unfortunately, while these bacteria can be important to us, they can also be harmful, if they get out of control. Often when we are ill a build up of bacteria can occur and some diseases are closely related to toxins and micro-organisms which build up in plaque in our mouths.

Like some of the greatest inventions, oil pulling is disarmingly simple as a technique. It simply involves swilling a small amount of oil around the gums and teeth. Little more than a teaspoon is required and this oil should be swilled and swished back and forth through the teeth and around the mouth. The process requires some patience, as fifteen to twenty minutes of this swilling is recommended. Gradually during this time the oil becomes a milky white and also becomes thinner in consistency. At this stage the oil should then be swilled back out of the mouth and the mouth then rinsed.

Simple enough? But what does it do? The oil, unlike toothpaste or mouthwash, adheres to the bacteria in the mouth. During the washing and swilling process the bacteria are captured in the oil and saliva; this is one of the reasons that the oil becomes milky white. Once the oil is ejected so are the bacteria. This not only removes excess bacteria very effectively but, in turn, inhibits the development of plaque which is caused by the bacteria normally present in the mouth. Oil pulling is one of the simplest and most effective ways of thoroughly cleansing your mouth, leaving it less liable to gum disease and tooth decay while at the same time helping to improve whiteness and tooth strength.

While this is great for your teeth it's also good news for you in general. There are, it is believed by many people, links between oil pulling and many other health conditions. In addition to the obvious benefits for your mouth and oral hygiene, conditions which may be helped, alleviated or avoided include;

- Dental problems including dental Cavities, Gingivitis, Gum Disease and abscesses

- Skin Problems, including acne, eczema and dermatitis

- Joint and bone conditions, including arthritis, joint pain and muscular pain or tension

Many other conditions have also been reported by those using the oil pulling technique to be alleviated or improved and these include migraine, colitis, diabetes, stomach ulcers, hypertension, periodontal disease and sinusitis. Even this list is not exhaustive and many practitioners believe that wider health benefits and resistance to disease can be achieved through the use of oil pulling.

Ayurvedic Traditions

Oil pulling is just one technique that has roots in the Ayurvedic Traditions of the Indian sub-continent. While in many western countries medical systems and practices have developed from knowledge rooted in the Classical era, Ayurvedic medicine and practices developed largely independently. Like other Eastern approaches to health and well-being, the tradition focuses on a more holistic approach to health. Ayurvedic medicine focuses on the whole body and on eating, exercising, meditating and cleanliness. While some 'alternative' traditions have been criticized for lack of scientific basis, Ayurvedic medicine is founded on some very practical principles.

Plant based medicines are a common feature of the tradition and the use of natural, wholesome and sustainable ingredients and elements strikes a chord with many people today. Oil pulling is one element of Ayurvedic practices and has been used for many centuries as an effective dental hygiene process and part of a wider approach to maintaining a healthy body.

Once only known in India and surrounding countries, Ayurvedic practices have become increasingly popular in recent years, as many health professionals recognize the need for a broader approach to health, rather than focusing on one particular issue. In addition, many traditional and alternative therapies focus more on prevention of ill health rather than curing or treating conditions as they arise. Oil pulling is a crucial part of a healthy lifestyle for many people, both in the practice's traditional homeland and much further afield.

Today, oil pulling has made the transition from alternative medicine to mainstream and widespread use.

The Basic Process

Oil pulling sounds simple at first but it does require some practice. The process involves taking a single teaspoon of oil – the different types of oil used are covered later in this book – and swilling it around the mouth for fifteen to twenty minutes. Most of us are familiar with swilling our mouths with a chemical based mouthwash after brushing but we normally only do this for a minute or so. Oil pulling is a longer process and takes some patience when first learning to correctly use the technique.

The swilling process does not have to be vigorous; simply swill the oil back and forth, between the teeth and around the gums, gently for up to twenty minutes. This process can be meditative in itself but it can be worth learning to quietly meditate during the oil pulling process. Meditation is now widely recognized even amongst modern clinical professionals as an important tool to achieving good health both physical and emotional. Adding oil pulling to your morning routine can encourage you to learn good meditation practices as well and incorporate these into your life at the same time.

Once the oil has whitened and thinned you can then spit it out into a sink or bowl (some people recommended disposing of used oil with trash, rather than adding it to the public sewer system). It's important to then rinse your mouth thoroughly with water; many people prefer distilled water as this will not introduce new bacteria into your mouth as soon as you have finished oil pulling!

Finally, brush and floss as normal. Oil pulling is believed to have an extremely positive effect on dental health but is not considered a substitute for your normal hygiene routine.

Chapter 2
Are You Sitting Comfortably?

Detailed Instructions for Effective Oil Pulling

The Oil Pulling process is simple, but as mentioned in the first chapter, it does take some practice. Once you get into the routine you'll find it's simple but making sure that you have time and space to complete a proper oil pulling session is important. Most of us have very busy lives these days and finding an extra twenty minutes in the day can be a challenge. Plan ahead and ensure that you have adequate time to put to one side – preferably first thing in the morning. Most practitioners emphasize that this is important and also that oil pulling should be conducted on an empty stomach.

During the night our bodies rest, recuperate and naturally process toxins. Also during the night the bacteria in our mouths are active – having built up during the previous day. Cleansing your mouth with oil pulling first thing in the day helps to eradicate harmful bacteria, toxins and pathogens which can adversely affect not only your dental health but your body in general.

Many people find that a sitting position is the best way to practice oil pulling. Ensure that you are comfortable, with your head slightly tilted backwards. Gently swill the oil around your mouth and relax your body while doing so. Some people choose to use relaxing music during the process while others simply sit quietly, enjoying the simple physical sensation of the cleaning process.

Practice makes Perfect

Although straightforward, it can be difficult to fully implement oil pulling straight away. The important thing to remember is that effective oil pulling takes time and patience. Don't become frustrated if you find that you want to finish after only five or ten minutes. Take things one step at a time and end each session when you are ready. At first this may mean that you are not able to complete the full twenty minutes but you'll find that remarkably quickly you are up to speed!

And Breathe

Relaxing while you are oil pulling is an essential part of the process and breathing in long, slow breaths through your nose is essential. Sometimes, until you are fully used to the technique, this can make you drowsy. Remember to stay alert, however, and do not swallow the oil! This is important, as is rinsing thoroughly after the session. The aim is, after all, to get those harmful bacteria and toxins out of your system, not further in!

Technical Tips

Gently push, pull, sip and suck the oil around your mouth and let it make its way between your teeth, into cavities and around your gums. The oil should gradually mix with your saliva and as it does so draw out bacteria and toxins. During the process enzymes are also activated in your saliva as it mixes with the oil. Many practitioners believe this helps to further draw out harmful toxins from the lining of the mouth and is, in part, responsible for the wider health benefits that oil pulling has to offer. Saliva is also generated during the process and with it's natural antiseptic effect helps to cleanse the gums, teeth and mouth and fighting any potential causes of infection. After twenty minutes the oil should have changed both color and consistency; becoming milky white and much thinner. If the oil remains yellow you will need to continue a little longer until it is thoroughly whitened. At this point it's time to spit and rinse.

Spit the oil into a sink a bowl to dispose of in the trash; then rinse your mouth thoroughly with water; distilled, bottled water is recommended as this is healthier and cleaner for your mouth. Finally brush, floss and use mouthwash as normal. This is important and shouldn't be forgotten. Oil pulling will remove many of the bacteria and substances in your mouth and will help to inhibit the build up of plaque but a final clean and floss is still important.

And Repeat?

In most cases oil pulling should be completed once a day, in the morning. However, there is no reason why you cannot complete the process again, two, three or four times throughout the day. The important factor is remember to complete each session before you eat and to ensure that you have time to complete a full twenty minute session. For those with loose teeth, gum disease or mouth ulcers and abscesses, multiple treatments each day have been found to be extremely effective at treating and alleviating these problems.

What to Expect

Oil pulling is remarkably effective at cleansing the teeth and mouth. Many converts to the technique notice whitening of the teeth in a very short space of time. In most cases a visible whitening effect begins to develop within two to four weeks. As the oil helps to reduce the build up of plaque, combined with brushing, it removes the bacteria that cause plaque in the first place and this effect becomes more noticeable over time.

For those with gum disease, or loose teeth, the results are commonly reported as rapid and startlingly effective. Gum strength is improved rapidly and teeth that were loose soon become firmly held in place. Those who suffer from bleeding gums will also notice a rapid improvement as bacteria are removed from the mouth, easing soreness and bleeding and helping to repair the structure of the gum. The combined effect of antiseptic qualities in the saliva produced during the oil pulling process, and the anti-inflammatory qualities of oils often used in the process, help to eradicate many different types of gum disease.

What many users of the technique love most of all is the low cost of oil pulling, compared to other dental hygiene techniques and also that all of this can be achieved without the need for chemicals or medication! In the next chapter we'll look a little more closely at how and why oil pulling is so effective at helping maintain a healthy mouth.

Chapter 3
A Controversial Topic

The Science behind the System

Although it has been around for longer than the modern dental industry, oil pulling has attracted both controversy and support from different quarters. Those who support the technique are often passionate about oil pulling and claim that it has a huge range of beneficial effects. Dentists and scientists have not always been wholly supportive of the technique. They have, however, admitted that whilst they are uncertain how effective oil pulling, is it is unlikely to have negative side effects.

However, some scientific studies have been undertaken in recent years and the results seem to offer support for oil pulling as an effective dental hygiene technique. There are a range of different oils used for oil pulling and these are looked at in more detail in the next chapter but one that seems to be not only popular with users but has been studied more closely is sesame oil. Sesame oil has proven qualities that can be beneficial to health and has been shown to reduce the bacteria and germ count in saliva and plaque. The science behind this is believed to be simply that lipids in the oil help to pull toxins, bacteria and germs out of the saliva and, at the same time, create a coating that makes the teeth resistant to these germs and bacteria.

Vested Interests?

Vegetable oils which are used in traditional techniques of oil pulling also contain emulsifiers and, mixed with saliva, this creates a 'soapy' effect. Although not tasting soapy, the mixture of oil and saliva is a natural cleansing agent and this is believed to be one of the main reasons that it is a perfect mixture to whiten teeth. While some dental experts doubt the efficacy of oil pulling the science behind the technique is very similar to the way in which soap was created in ancient times. Animal fats, as well as vegetable fats, are combined with water and chemicals to create soap. In today's modern industrial processes this is done on a large scale, using all manner of unpleasant chemicals. While it may not suit all dentists (or the manufacturers of mass-produced dental products) to support a cheaper, more natural home-produced product, there's little reason scientifically why it should be less effective.

Plaque Busting

Plaque is a thin film made up of a combination of food scraps, mucus and bacteria. It builds up in layers over time around the base of your teeth - between them and in hard to reach pockets. Many of the components that make up plaque are perfectly natural and some bacteria are essential for good oral health. Plaque is really a by-product of the mouth functioning properly. However, it can also cause problems as it provides a great home for bacteria and can also hold chemicals and pesticides in the mouth, along with additives from food. Plaque build up in pockets that are hard to access when brushing can lead to gum damage and corrosion or cavities in the teeth. While regular brushing, flossing and dental check ups all go a long way to removing plaque, none will easily clear the hidden pockets of plaque and bacteria that do the most damage to our teeth and gums. This is where oil pulling is believed to have a very beneficial effect in terms of oral hygiene. The slow process allows the oil to thoroughly penetrate gaps, cavities and other hiding places where difficult to reach plaque builds up. The oil and saliva mixture adhere to bacteria and plaque in these awkward, inaccessible spaces and remove it.

The Wider Implications

While the sticky consistency of the oil, the combination of emulsifiers and saliva, the toxin absorbing effects of the oil pulling process all go a long way to explaining how effective it is as a dental hygiene technique, it's less easy to understand just how oil pulling can help with a number of other illnesses. Some of the oils used in the process do themselves contain a number of positive health benefits. From antibacterial to anti-inflammatory qualities many also contain important antioxidants, enzymes and vitamins. Some are believed to help with cell regeneration both in the mouth and the body in general. Oils can be combined with a number of other essential oils to create a 'flavor' but also to take advantage of proven positive health effects that natural plant extracts contain. Ayurvedic medicine is based very much on the use of plants and plant extracts and, although not all multinationals would be happy to admit it, many widely used medicines use surprisingly natural ingredients thanks to their proven health benefits.

Life in a Slower Lane?

Another simple factor that is often overlooked when it comes to using the oil pulling technique is the thoroughness of the process and the pace at which it is completed. Many of us live our lives in a rush, today, and a quick brush and floss may not always be the best way to thoroughly cleanse our mouths! Oil pulling is a much slower process, a relaxed process and one that means a very thorough mouth cleansing result. Unlike our super-fast modern habits it's one that is based on time, showing a little respect for our bodies and giving them space to work in conjunction with natural elements.

Chapter 4 – Oily Solutions

Oils to Use in Oil Pulling

Oil pulling can be completed using a number of different oils. The best type of oil to use is food-grade, unrefined oil produced using a cold-press technique. Most practitioners prefer to use organically produced oils which are easy to source from both health food and mainstream stores. Organic, cold-pressed oils are the purest form of natural vegetable oils available on the market and are ideal for oil pulling, as they contain no additives. This is an important consideration, as the process is designed to remove toxins from your system – not add them!

Your Choice

Personal choice is often a big factor in deciding which oil to use for oil pulling and can depend on taste as much as anything else. The most commonly used oils are sesame oil, avocado oil, coconut and olive oil. Sunflower and safflower oils are also popular and while the general effect of each oil is the same, some have additional qualities that make them popular with those using oil pulling on a regular basis. Additionally, some people like to add essential oils to the main oil partly for flavor but mainly for potential additional health benefits and qualities available from these oils. In this chapter we'll look at the main oils and their specific qualities.

Sesame Oil

This oil has been used for hundreds, probably thousands, of years by healers and health practitioners. While early users may not have understood the science behind the effectiveness of sesame oil, modern science has been able to shed light on the real benefits of sesame oil for good health. Naturally both antiviral and anti-fungal it's an excellent oil to use for oil pulling. Sesame oil has also been found to have antioxidant properties which, when used in oil pulling, may explain some of the wider positive health benefits of the technique. Sesame oil is quickly absorbed by the skin (or lining of the mouth) and helps to reduce damage to cells that can result from the oxidization process. Although a natural process, oxidization can result in chain reactions within the cells of plants and animals (us included) which cause cell damage, resulting in changes in the body and potential ill health. Antioxidants inhibit the oxidization process helping to reduce the risks of negative changes in the body's cells. For those with existing medical conditions reducing oxidization is important. The immune system is often focused on dealing with a specific condition and needs the help of antioxidants to reduce the oxidization process. The changes in cells that oxidization causes are responsible for a massive number of conditions, including development of cancer, stroke and heart disease. Sesame oil is, therefore, an excellent choice for oil pulling with numerous beneficial side effects.

Coconut Oil

Long associated with the beauty industry, coconut oil has also long been used in a medicinal setting. For oil pulling it ranks along with sesame oil as an excellent choice for many of the same reasons. It has antibacterial, antiviral and antioxidant properties, and all of the associated benefits described above. Chemically, coconut oil has a simple composition and is easily absorbed by the body. Our body is able to metabolize the nutritional components of coconut oil extremely efficiently and the oil and other coconut products are considered useful for weight-loss. Coconut provides energy and contains fats and nutrients that are processed by the body contributing to important factors in the body's processes which include bone strength and joint health. Coconut oil (and other coconut products) are considered high in fat, by some, but these fats are healthy fats that do not contribute to weight gain or heart disease – in fact reducing the dangers of both! One reason that coconut oil is popular for oil pulling is also that the taste is pleasant! It's a small consideration, but one that many find important; the oil is sweet, mild and gentle, making it an easy oil to spend twenty minutes or so a day with!

Olive Oil

This is easily sourced from major stores and that may be one reason why it is so popular for oil pulling. The chances are that you have some in your kitchen already and it can be a great (cost-effective) choice. Olive is considered to be a healthy oil for culinary purposes and is believed to reduce the risks of developing some cancers and help to reduce cholesterol levels. The chemical make up of the oil also includes an anti-inflammatory component and (as with sesame and coconut) it has powerful antioxidant properties. Then there's the taste! And that is the big problem for many people in using olive oil for oil pulling. Of the options, olive oil, can be the least attractive on the taste-bud sensation front! If you happen to love the taste, then olive oil can be a great option. If not, it's likely to put you off the idea completely, very early on in your efforts. Olive has the same advantages of other oils and is also, in many cases, the most cost effective solution. However, if it's a taste that you can't learn to love then you may find that other oils are for you.

Sunflower Oil

This is one of the most traditional oils used in oil pulling within the Ayurvedic traditions. Not only does it have proven health properties similar to sesame oil but it also contains high levels of vitamin E. This is a vitamin found in many health products and is often found in skin moisturizers and creams aimed at improving skin related conditions including eczema and dermatitis. Sunflower oil is recommended for those looking to reduce cholesterol and is believed to help those suffering from arthritis. In terms of flavor, the oil is mild and one that many people find pleasant for both oil pulling and for culinary uses.

Avocado Oil

This is an oil that is increasingly popular for those who require a cholesterol-lowering alternative in their diets. The oil has low levels of saturated fats and has proven beneficial at reducing cholesterol, while also containing high levels of vitamin E, essential for cell growth, repair and healthy development and well documented for reducing the risk of coronary disease. On a taste level, like coconut oil, this is a popular choice for many. In an oil pulling context, avocado oil is an excellent choice offering wide-ranging benefits, although it may be more difficult to source in some locations and may prove to be one of the more expensive options for this reason.

Important Considerations

- Flavor will play a part and it's important to choose an oil that you find palatable. While olive oil is widely available it's not always a favorite for oil pulling. The main oils, sesame, coconut and olive all have similar health benefits and are equally beneficial in terms of oil pulling.

- One of the most significant factors to remember is that unrefined, cold-pressed and organic oils are the ones to use. Mechanically produced oils will normally contain other ingredients and non-organically produce oils may contain more toxins than they remove! Although slightly more expensive, it's important to remember that the oil pulling process is designed to improve your health (oral and general) and it's worth the additional cost for the best quality oils.

- Some people prefer to use one or several different oils for the oil pulling process. Alternating between different oils each day can be a good way to gain additional benefits from the different oils and it also, simply, introduces some variety into the technique.

- Depending on your specific health needs, choosing an oil which best addresses any existing health conditions also makes sense. For those with persistent or recurring gum disease, for example the anti-inflammatory qualities of olive oil can be very helpful, while coconut oil will also combat bacteria and infection in the gums.

Chapter 5

Happy, Healthy Mouths

The Benefits for Oral Health

The most obvious benefits of oil pulling relate to oral health. The general condition of your teeth and gums is not only important in itself but can also be an indicator of, or a cause of, wider health issues.   Sore gums, yellowed teeth and bleeding when brushing can all be a sign of gum disease and the presence of too much bacteria in your mouth.   They can also be side-effects of other conditions, ranging from heart disease to kidney problems. White, shining teeth and strong, healthy pink gums are a sign that your mouth, and health in general, is in great shape.

However, the very basic point of oil pulling is to maintain a healthy mouth and this is the starting point for many of those attracted to the technique. This chapter looks in more detail at the effect that oil pulling has in terms of oral and dental health and hygiene.

Rapid Reactions

In a matter of weeks, most people who take up oil pulling as a technique notice that their teeth are whiter and that loose teeth (a sign of problems with the gum) begin to show signs of firming up. Certainly, this is the case within around four to six weeks but many individuals report that signs of improvement appear within a week to ten days. If you already have a high standard of oral and dental hygiene it's likely that effects will be subtle but improvements will occur and these will occur quickly. For those with persistent, or historic, problems with both the teeth and gums it may take longer – but persevere as results will develop in a surprisingly short time. Oil will reach into those difficult to access parts of the mouth, between the teeth and in nooks and crannies not normally reached by simple brushing and even flossing. The action of the oil on bacteria and toxins that have built up over time is relatively quick to produce results and will start to have a beneficial effect, reducing bleeding when brushing, removing plaque, staining and improving health rapidly. Most people report that from the start their mouths feel much cleaner after using oil pulling and that even their sense of taste begins to improve.

Tooth Decay and Oil Pulling

Most dentists will argue that the only way to resolve cavities is to either remove the offending tooth or to fill the cavity – depending on the extent of the damage. However, oil pulling will not only help to prevent tooth decay but may even help to reverse it. This is a fairly astounding claim to many people – especially those who make a living as dentists!

Cavities and decay are the result of acid produced in the mouth by bacteria that inhabit it. While some bacteria are necessary for good oral health, our modern diets and lifestyles can quickly lead to an overabundance of bacteria. Diets which contain higher levels of sugars and fats – often found in the types of meals that we regularly consume – provide a feast for not only us but our resident bacteria. These organisms produce higher levels of acid when exposed to regular high doses of their favorite sugary foods. The result is the increase in dental decay.

Our bodies, having evolved over many millennium, have already developed strategies to deal with bacteria in the mouth. The saliva that we produce is designed to fight infection and injury in the mouth and also to neutralize acid and to flush it away. Oil pulling works alongside saliva in two important ways; firstly it increases the production of saliva during the process, which helps to attack the acid levels in the mouth. Secondly, the oil is attractive to the bacteria, which get caught up in it, helping to remove them.

Where cavities are beginning to develop this is extremely useful. Minerals contained within the saliva can help to re-coat areas that are beginning to show signs of damage. For this reason, oil pulling appears to be an effect way to not only combat cavities and tooth decay, by helping to remove bacteria and neutralize acid, but by encouraging higher levels of saliva and the consequent deposit of minerals on weak areas of the tooth's surface.

Halitosis

Bad breath; it's never a pleasant subject and, for those who suffer from more severe cases it can be very distressing indeed. Halitosis is usually caused by more serious forms of gum disease, including gingivitis and periodontitis. It can also be a side-effect of other conditions, including diabetes. Apart from the unpleasant physical aspects of bad breath, many sufferers can experience shyness, low self-esteem and become withdrawn, depressed or anxious. In general, this creates stress – which is never good for our health – and usually has a negative effect on your health, often making matters worse.

The cause of halitosis is, again, those irritating bacteria that build up in our mouths. With conditions like gingivitis, the build up of bacteria is rapid and, apart from damage to gums, nearly always involves a level of bad breath. General dentistry options for halitosis include mouthwashes containing chemicals that kill off the bacteria. Many people also rely on sprays that disguise bad breath. Both techniques work reasonably well but oil pulling addresses the basic cause of the problem. While mouthwash does kill off bacteria in the short-term it doesn't (unfortunately) stem the tide. Oil pulling, however, reduces the number of bacteria each time you use the technique and on a daily basis simply removes the bacteria responsible for the bad smell. Used daily, on a regular and ongoing basis, this means that oil pulling will have extremely rapid and positive effects on conditions like halitosis. Additionally, compared to medical solutions, it's less costly and, importantly, doesn't involve using chemicals which many people are reluctant to use as they produce unwanted side-effects.

Gum Disease

Swelling, inflamed, sore and often bleeding gums are a sign of tissue damage and decay. Gum problems can be short term or long term and some people suffer from recurrent bouts of gum disease throughout their lives. Stress can increase the risk of gum disease, as can the consumption of sugary, fatty foods. Gums that are in poor condition can also be the result of other illnesses and the main problem is that once tissue damage begins it can lead to other problems within the mouth, including loose teeth and the development of ulcers and abscesses.

Gingivitis is a term covering this type of damage to the tissue of the gums and, left untreated, it can lead to serious problems. Many cases are mild and are only indicated by the presence of a little blood on the bristles of your tooth brush. This can come and go at different times but left untreated there is the danger that it will develop into a more serious infection. Often the condition occurs as the result of other illnesses or conditions and is not uncommon during pregnancy, when our bodies have a lot of other issues to deal with! Poor dental hygiene is one very common cause and gingivitis can also develop as a reaction to some common medicines.

Oil pulling for gingivitis has been shown to be highly effective in a number of studies. It reduces the level of gingivitis and bacteria that are behind the disease. Gingivitis is caused by microbes in plaque and oil pulling effectively removes these microbes along with helping to reduce the longer term build up of the plaque, helping on two levels to resolve problems with the gums.

Health Gums, Healthy Teeth and Brighter Smiles all Round

By removing bacteria, which are responsible for plaque deposits, creating acidity in the mouth and causing gingivitis and other gum disease, oil pulling is a proven and effective technique to improve your oral and dental health. By encouraging the development of healthy gums it can allow gum tissues and ligaments the space to grow, increase in health and support strong teeth. In general oil pulling helps to improve overall health, reduce any cases of loose teeth and can even have a positive anti-cavity effect. It also encourages the body's natural techniques for maintaining a healthy environment in the mouth, attacking the causes of cavities and decay and helping restore any damaged areas to a much healthier state.

Chapter 6

Not Just For Your Mouth!

Oil Pulling and Associated Health Benefits

While oil pulling has obvious benefits for dental and oral health there are many claims made about its effectiveness at treating, or reducing the risk of developing, many other illnesses. Skeptics argue that oil pulling is unlikely to be an effective technique in a broader context of good health, while those who favor the technique are strongly convinced that oil pulling is a powerful way in which to combat many serious conditions.

There has, as yet, been limited scientific research conducted into oil pulling and some of the claims its adherents make in relation to wider health. There are, however, some studies which support the basic principles which appear to be in operation in the oil pulling process. In addition, there is much to support these claims by way of anecdotal evidence. While the subject deserves more in-depth study, on a scientific basis, there is considerable agreement that the practice is not in any way detrimental to health or dangerous in itself. While the scientific community remain skeptical, they do largely agree that oil pulling is not a risky technique. For those with a number of serious conditions it's important to continue to seek traditional medical support, advice and treatment but oil pulling has, for many people, provided an additional way in which to combat illness and disease.

Heart Disease

Improvement and technological advances in science, industry, manufacturing and technology have led to great leaps forward in many countries around the world. They have changed the way we live and have had massively positive impacts on public health. Traditional illnesses, responsible for many deaths in the past, have been all but eradicated. However, in their place there are new threats that are, in part, down to the changes in our method of living, working and playing. Heart disease is a huge problem across the Western world, where our diets have improved but our lives have become more sedentary.

Traditional diets, more exercise and simpler ways of living are all good ways to combat the risk of developing heart disease. While claims that oil pulling may have a positive effect on heart disease are viewed with skepticism by some people, the simple science behind the claim bears some scrutiny. All of the oils used in the technique have strong antibacterial properties and these properties target the bacteria like streptococcus which causes inflammation. Inflammation of the muscles around the heart and the arteries are significant contributing factors to heart disease, stroke, high blood pressure and related conditions. While medical confirmation is not widely available that oil pulling can reduce problems relating to these conditions, there is a growing body of evidence to suggest that reduction in inflammatory substances within the body is extremely beneficial for people with these conditions and can, of course, help to reduce the risk of developing heart disease.

Migraine

The simple fact with migraine and oil pulling is that Ayurvedic practitioners have, for centuries, considered it a basic method for treatment and prevention of migraine and severe headache. For those who suffer from migraine, another simple factor is that if there's a chance oil pulling can help it's got to be worth a try! Migraine can be hugely debilitating;

leading to a crippling condition which includes vomiting, sensitivity to light and severe pain. Some migraine sufferers only display mild symptoms but those who live with frequent moderate to severe symptoms can find that their ability to conduct a normal life is badly affected. Traditional painkillers, or specially prescribed ones, can have some affect but even these do not always deal with migraine sufficiently. The real causes behind migraine are not clearly understood by the scientific and medical communities and treatments vary in efficacy for different individuals.

Oil pulling adherents believe that there is a strong link between toxins that we ingest and migraine. This has significant basis in fact. Many sufferers find that migraines are triggered by certain foods; wine, processed foods, mono-sodium-glutamate and a whole range of additives commonly found in many food products. Added to this environmental pollutants – cigarettes, cleaning products and exhaust or manufacturing fumes - all contain toxins which have been linked to increase occurrence of migraines. Oil pulling is a technique which helps to eliminate both bacteria and toxins from the body. It has been shown that using the technique helps to rid toxins from the mouth and skin, by absorption into lining of the mouth, simply gathering these toxins up in the liquid and then helping to expel them from the body. Increased enzyme activity and production also occurs during the process and these enzymes have a strong anti-toxin effect.

One additional element to the process, along with the removal of the toxins, is the meditative quality of the technique, which helps to reduce stress. Ultimately, in the case of migraines, many practitioners have found it is one of the most effective techniques for stopping migraines occurring in the first place, while also being helpful at reducing symptoms during the early stages of an attack.

Joint and Bone Pain and Conditions

Oil is essential for the body in order to help lubricate joints, bones and build strong healthy muscles. This has been recognized for many centuries in many medical traditions around the world and is strongly supported by modern day science. Swelling around the joints and bones is normally caused by a build up of fluids and is the result of a variety of different conditions. It can be caused by an injury – a broken bone or torn ligament, Fluid builds up to protect the damaged area but also causes soreness and difficulty in movement. Swelling and inflammation is also caused by a range of diseases which damage the bone; arthritis is one of the more common diseases in which inflammation becomes pronounced and painful.

Oil pulling has been proven to reduce inflammation, simply by virtue of the fact that the oils used have natural anti-inflammatory properties. Apart from vegetable oils, cod-liver oil is a well known supplement effective at strengthening bones, joints and tendons. Using the oil pulling technique helps to reduce inflammation and remove toxins and bacteria from the body. During the process many of the essential nutritional elements and vitamins within the oil are ingested directly through the lining of the mouth and it's this aspect of oil pulling which is believed to be responsible for its positive affects on a whole range of joint, bone and muscular related injuries and diseases.

Sleep and Insomnia

Good sleep is essential for health and recent studies have linked sleep disorders to many major diseases. From heart disease to cancer, the list of illnesses which can be potentially triggered by poor sleep patterns seems endless. Again, modern lifestyles can be a major issue in disrupting our sleep pattern. With an "always on" attitude to life and widespread use of non-natural light, major research is now showing that our natural body clock is severely disrupted by our way of life. One important function of sleep is the detoxification that our bodies conduct overnight. Suffering from disrupted, or poor sleep, inhibits the body's natural processes which can lead to a range of short and longer term problems.

Most evidence that oil pulling has a positive effect on poor or disrupted sleeping patterns is anecdotal. Many people who use the technique, and have previously had sleep problems, have found that, unexpectedly, their sleeping patterns improve radically. It seems possible that oil pulling, by removing toxins, assists the body to process these toxins, requiring less effort during the night and leaving the body to rest more fully. Other supporters of oil pulling have suggested that it is possible that antioxidants contained in oil help to improve the function of our glands. This may account for improved sleep as melatonin, which is responsible for sleep regulation, is produced by our endocrine system. Antioxidants play an important role in the healthy functioning of many of our major organs and improved health in the whole body is one important factor in the promotion of healthy sleep. Although further studies are required, it is certainly possible that there are very clear links between oil pulling and improving the quality of our sleep pattern.

Stress

Stress and depression have a huge impact on our health in general. Our state of mind is directly linked to our physical health – if you've ever noticed how you feel physically sick when hearing bad news you'll already be aware of how mental and physical ill health are directly linked. Modern science has linked stress to many physical illnesses and stress has a clear and direct impact on coronary health. It is also now widely recognized to have a major link to the development of many cancers.

When we become stressed our bodies produce a high level of a number of hormones. Adrenalin and cortisol are two hormones produced to deal with stress. During the production of these hormones our immune system is temporarily shut down – in order to stop the body attacking these substances. Often cortisol floods our system and while this is present our natural immunity is compromised. Oil pulling can help to reduce the amount of cortisol in our system (the hormone is deposited in the mouth in saliva). Oil adheres to the hormones within the saliva and these are expelled at the end of the process. By reducing the period of time between the 'deployment' of cortisol and adrenalin, and removing them from our system oil pulling helps to switch the immune system back on and get our bodies functioning as normal again.

Keep taking the tablets?

While the benefits of oil pulling are widely supported by many users and healers around the world, it's important to continue to seek medical supervision for any existing illnesses. There seems to be a very strong scientific basis for many of the benefits of the oil pulling technique and as has been shown many times in the past, traditional techniques often become endorsed by scientists and clinicians when they have been more thoroughly tested and researched.

Chapter 7
Time to start?

Oil Pulling Process Summary

So, if you've read this far and feel that oil pulling is a technique that you can't afford not to try, it's time to get started! Remember these important points as you begin to use oil pulling to improve your oral health and increase your overall health.

- Use cold-pressed, organically produced oils of high quality.

- Pick an oil that suits your taste and (using this book) one that addresses any specific concerns. The best oils to use are; sunflower, olive, coconut, avocado and, in particular, sesame oil.

- Use a single teaspoon of oil first thing in the morning on an empty stomach.

- Relax, meditate and take your time, oil pulling should be practiced for about twenty minutes.

- When oil and saliva have mixed and eliminated bacteria and toxins the mixture will be thinner and milky white.

- Once you're done rinse your mouth thoroughly with water – distilled water is best.

- Brush, floss and use mouthwash as normal, it's still important to continue with your normal dental routine in addition to oil pulling.

Sit back, relax and watch the results begin to show. Remember, the technique can take a little practice, so don't get frustrated at first. Practice makes perfect and you'll soon learn to incorporate a relaxing, meditative twenty minutes into your morning routine. Your teeth should become clearly whiter within a matter of weeks and a number of health improvements will often begin to develop quickly as well. When your friends and family start to question you enviously, don't forget to share the secret of your new, low-cost, simple oral hygiene routine!

Conclusion

Thank you again for downloading this book!

I hope this book was extremely informative on the entire process of oil pulling. Make sure to refer to this book again and again for any questions you may have!

The next step is to go out and get the oil of your choice from your local health food store and implement this in your weekly routine. Like any new habit, start slowly and you will be getting the immense rewards of this ancient process before you know it!

Finally, if you enjoyed this book, please take the time to share your thoughts and post a review on Amazon. I would really appreciate it!

Thank you again for spending some time with me!

Your Friend,

Ashley Stone

Preview Of 'Coconut Oil Hacks'

What is Coconut Oil?

Coconut oil is natural, edible oil which is extracted from the fruit of the coconut palm tree. The oil is nearly colorless with a white tint. Coconut oil is thicker than most fats. While it is technically a liquid, some varieties appear to be solid. This can be attributed to its high saturated fat content. When stored properly, coconut oil can last up to two years before going rancid.

It is considered both an emollient, a surfactant, and a lubricant. Coconut oil has found countless applications, many of them related to nutrition, weight-loss, skin care, disease prevention, and hygiene. Careful studies have discovered antibacterial, antimicrobial, antioxidant, and anti-fungal qualities to validate its wide range of uses.

History

Historical records show that coconut palms has been used as a medicine and source of nutrition for at least 3960 years. Throughout that time, the coconut has been seen as a sustainable resource for fruit, water, milk, and oil. Coconut and its extracted oil have been widely used in tropical locations around the globe including Polynesia, Micronesia, South America, Africa, Central America, Asia, and Melanesia.

Some of the most detailed accounts related to the use of coconut oil as a medicine belong to the Ayurveda healing tradition. Ancient documents confirm that Ayurveda began making use of coconut oil as early as 1500 BC. One famous earlyEuropean explorer, Captain Cook, recorded his observations of the Pacific natives, including the prevalent use of coconut oil.

WWII medics found themselves in desperate need of saline to save the lives of allied soldiers. It was not long before they learned that the water of unripe coconuts made an excellent substitute. After the war, soldiers brought their appreciation for the coconut home with them. Soon coconut oil became a popular staple. It was sold as margarine in the United Kingdom, and as "coconut butter" in the United States.

Unfortunately, the popularity of coconut oil would see a sharp declined in 1954. At that time, the United States was fighting a rise in coronary heart disease. David Kritchevsky published two academic papers which discussed the relationships between cholesterol levels and blocked arteries. He also praised polyunsaturated fats as a better choice for heart disease prevention. Coconut oil, with its naturally high saturated fat content, was cast aside. For decades it would continue to be shunned by both doctors and nutritionists.

Fortunately, modern research has brought a new light to misconceptions of the past. While coconut oil contains saturated fat, it is clearly different from other natural fats and oils. It can actually help lower overall cholesterol levels. Additionally, it carries essential antibacterial and antiviral properties. This new information has come at a time when the world is searching for inexpensive, natural, and sustainable sources of healthy lipids. Its countless uses are again being recognized. Coconut oil is now being added to diets and used to stimulate healing.

To read more of Coconut Oil Hacks:
go to: **http://amzn.to/1nB8MPo**

Printed in Great Britain
by Amazon